Autophagy

The Key To Living Long, Healthy, and Happy!

By Erik Smith

Table of Contents

Free Stuff

Do you want to get notified when I have free books? Then sign up for my newsletter. I will never spam you. I will only send you valuable stuff that you can use to help you improve your life.

Sign up here - http://forms.aweber.com/form/26/1968511626.htm

Disclaimer

This document is geared towards providing exact and reliable information in regards to the topic and issue covered. The publication is sold with the idea that the publisher is not required to render accounting, officially permitted, or otherwise, qualified services. If advice is necessary, legal or professional, a practiced individual in the profession should be ordered.

- From a Declaration of Principles which was accepted and approved equally by a Committee of the American Bar Association and a Committee of Publishers and Associations.

The information herein is offered for informational purposes solely, and is universal as so. The presentation of the information is without contract or any type of guarantee assurance.

The trademarks that are used are without any consent, and the publication of the trademark is without permission or backing by the trademark owner. All trademarks and brands within this book are for clarifying purposes only and are the owned by the owners themselves, not affiliated with this document.

Introduction

This book aims to enhance your understanding of autophagy. It gives you relevant information to give you a better appreciation of autophagy and how it helps the body to function optimally.

The book contains concrete strategies about how to induce the condition. It provides concrete and specific instructions on what you can do to promote autophagy.

The book explains how fasting may be the best strategy for inducing autophagy. It outlines the different intermittent fasting strategies. It goes into detail about how to apply the strategies in your daily life.

With detailed instructions at your fingertips, you can choose which strategy works well for your lifestyle. You can even develop your own strategy by combining two or more of the techniques that the book provides.

After reading this book, I hope that you will be able to use what you have learned to achieve your long-term health goals.

Thanks again for downloading this book, I hope you enjoy it!

What Is Autophagy?

The body goes through a lot of metabolic processes. As a result, cells (or some of their parts) get damaged. This is normal. Some factors like aging, stress and the onslaught of free radicals can result to even greater damage.

Senescent cells are cells that remain in the organs and tissues, but serve no real purpose.

When damaged and senescent cells stay in the body, they tend to activate inflammatory pathways. Your immune system becomes weaker. You become an easy target for a wide range of diseases.

Autophagy is a process that helps the body get rid of damaged and senescent cells.

The word "autophagy" is a combination of the Greek words "auto'" which means self, and "phagy," which means eating. It refers to the body's natural metabolic process of eating its own tissue, especially when the body is starved or ill.

Autophagy is a survival mechanism. It is the body's way of responding to stress and protecting itself.

In recent years, researchers have discovered that autophagy can prevent the early signs of aging. It appears to also have a wide range of benefits for the immune system, the nervous system, the cardiovascular system, and metabolism in general.

By "eating itself," the body promotes the renewal of healthy cells. It destroys and eliminates damaged components found inside cells. It reuses the waste matter that cells produce and builds new material for the repair and regeneration of new cells.

Autophagy helps the body "clean up." It makes the body stronger. It enables the body to fight stress and diseases.

What Are the Benefits of Autophagy?

Simply put, autophagy promotes health at the cellular level. It is a mechanism for health and self-preservation. It helps the body to clean, recycle, and regenerate new and healthy cells so that the body regains optimal function.

Here's a quick rundown of what autophagy does for the body:

•   Autophagy provides energy and molecular building blocks for cells.

•   It helps recycle damaged proteins and other cell tissues to rebuild the cells.

•   It helps cells produce usable energy from oxygen and nutrients.

•   It helps the cells eliminate toxic substances.

•   It makes DNA more stable.

•   It keeps organs and tissues healthy by protecting the healthy cells and getting rid of harmful or diseased ones.

•   It has the potential for preventing or delaying neurodegenerative illnesses like Alzheimer's disease.

•   It protects the nervous system and improves cognitive function by promoting the growth of healthy nerve cells.

•   It protects the body from heart disease.

•   It helps the immune system function more efficiently.

•   It reduces inflammation.

•   It slows down aging.

•   It helps with digestive health.

- It prevents cancer.

- It helps you manage your weight.

- It helps prevent heart disease, liver problems, diabetes, cancer, and other chronic health problems.

What Can You Do to Stimulate Autophagy?

All cells go through natural autophagy. They tend to go through more actively when they are under stress or become deprived of nutrients.

You can induce autophagy. You can increase the stressors. You can also deliberately do things to deprive the body of nutrients.

Physical exercise is a "good stressor." Fasting, on the other hand, is a temporary way to restrict calories and deprive the body of nutrients. Both have been identified as effective strategies for inducing autophagy. It is interesting to note that both exercise and calorie-restriction are approaches often recommended to control weight, delay aging, and inhibit a variety of age-associated illnesses.

1. Practice Fasting

There is a number of things you can do to induce autophagy. Foremost among them are changing lifestyle habits and going on a diet.

Studies show that the best thing you can do is to go on a fast.

There is nothing complicated about fasting. You simply stop eating (or severely limit your food intake) for a specified period of time. You go without food, although you can still take water, tea, or coffee.

IMF or Intermittent Fasting is a dietary strategy that has become quite popular. It generates serious interest because people who practice it seem to enjoy many health benefits as a result of the diet.

Here is a quick look at how fasting works:

Intermittent fasting is a strategy where you eat only during specific periods of time. You have several options about how to do this.

You can practice alternate day fasting. On a fasting day, you limit yourself to having 1 or 2 meals that only contain around 500 calories. This will severely cut down the number of calories you take in. On a non-fasting day, you don't set any limit to what you eat. This basically means that you eat one day and fast on the next day.

You can also set an "eating window." You limit your eating to 4 to 8 hours and fast for the other 16 to 20 hours.

What form of fasting works best for autophagy?

Health care experts say that fasting between 24 to 48 hours can give you the strongest results. However, most people find it difficult to go without food for such a relatively long period of time.

An easier option is to go without eating for between 12 and 36 hours at a time. You abstain from eating in between meals and stick to 1 or 2 nutrient-dense meals a day. Have your last meal between 6 and 7 at night and break your fast at 7 in the morning. If you can manage it, skip breakfast and have brunch between 11 and 12 noon. This schedule extends your fasting period and brings faster results.

Once your stomach gets used to going without meals, you can go on occasional 2-to-3 day fasts.

2. Go on a Keto Diet

Ketosis is a metabolic state characterized by the production of ketones. Ketosis is great for losing weight. It gives your body a stable supply of energy. You'll have greater focus and concentration. It produces a feeling of satiety that results in less hunger pangs and food cravings.

The fastest way to achieve ketosis is by not eating anything (or going on a fast). An easier way to achieve ketosis is to go on a keto diet.

The keto or ketogenic diet brings results similar to those that you get from fasting.

It is a low-carb, high-fat diet. You eat a lot of rich and fatty food and restrict your intake of carbohydrates.

When you go on a ketogenic diet, you choose your food carefully. 75% of your daily calories should come from fat and only 5 to 10% should come from carbohydrates.

A keto diet includes substantial amounts of olive oil, high-fat coconut oil, butter, ghee (a semi-fluid clarified butter popular in South Asian cooking), fermented cheese, meat, seeds, nuts, and avocado. It also includes fiber-rich vegetables so you can fill your requirements for antioxidants and vitamins.

Normally, your body gets its energy from glucose, a form of sugar that comes from carbohydrates. When there isn't enough glucose available, the body turns to fat for fuel.

The ketogenic diet gets its name from the word "keto." This is because the diet makes the body produce ketones – small molecules that are used for fuel.

Ketones are an alternative source of energy. When the body uses up its supply of glucose (which is its principal source of energy), it turns to ketones to provide the fuel.

The body produces ketones on a ketogenic diet. The diet includes very limited amount of carbohydrates, protein in moderation, and a great degree of fatty food.

The liver uses fat to produce ketones. When you go on a keto diet, your body switches from glucose to fat as its fuel source. It burns fat the entire time. When insulin levels decrease, the body burns fat faster. It turns to stored fat and burns them off.

What to Eat and Avoid on a Ketogenic Diet

What to Eat

A ketogenic nutritional plan is built around the following foods:

- Mackerel tuna, trout, salmon, and other fatty fish

- Turkey, chicken, ham, bacon, sausage, steak, and other red meat

- Omega 3 whole eggs or pastured eggs

- Grass-fed cream and butter

- Almonds, flax seeds, walnuts, chia seeds, pumpkin seeds, and other seeds and nuts

- Avocado oil, coconut oil, olive oil (preferably extra virgin), and other healthy oils

- Mozzarella, blue, goat, cheddar, cream, and other unprocessed cheese

- Guacamole, preferably freshly made, and whole avocados

- Peppers, onions, tomatoes, green leafy vegetables, and other low-carb veggies

- Spices, pepper, salt, healthy herbs, and other similar condiments

What to Avoid

Limit foods that are high in carbs. Reduce your intake of (or eliminate) the following foods from your diet:

- Candy, cake, ice-cream, fruit juice, soda, and other sugary foods

- Cereal, pasta, rice, wheat-based products, and other starches or grains

- Parsnips, carrots, sweet potatoes, potatoes, and other tubers and root vegetables

- All fruit except strawberries and other berries (but only in very small portions)

- Chickpeas, lentils, kidney beans, peas, and other legumes or beans

- Diet products and other low-fat products which are usually carbs-rich and highly processed

- Sauces or condiments that are sweet

- Mayonnaise, highly processed vegetable oils and other unhealthy fats

- Alcoholic beverages (because of their high carb content)

3. Get Regular Physical Exercise

Physical exercise is recognized as a good stressor. It induces autophagy, especially in the pancreas, liver, muscles, adipose tissues, and other organs involved in the regulation of metabolism.

Exercise helps break down tissues, and repair and regenerate them.

Is it all right to exercise while you are fasting?

Doing this may take some getting used to, especially when you haven't exercised for a long time. Once you get used to fasting and see the results, however, you may even feel more motivated to exercise.

While all forms of exercise induce autophagy, experts suggest that you include a few minutes of intense aerobic exercise in your program. Half an hour of intense cardiovascular exercise can cause autophagy in the heart and skeletal muscle tissues.

High-Intensity Interval Training or HIIT appears to be the best form of exercise to induce autophagy. It brings you to a sweet spot for good stress. It applies the right degree of stress to elicit biochemical change.

HIIT is built around the short-term high-level stress concept. Using an HIIT exercise program (resistance training and weightlifting) for 30 minutes every other day helps you give autophagy a strong boost.

You can use the same concept for other forms of exercise. If you are fond of walking, you can alternate brisk walking and slower-pace walking to achieve similar results.

4.   Get enough sleep.

Sleep has restorative benefits.

If you sleep better, you tend to look younger, feel more energetic, and live longer.

Your circadian rhythm (or your daily wake/sleep cycles) has an effect on autophagy. If you are able to get quality rest and sleep, you trigger autophagy. You help activate your body's natural recycling program.

On the other hand, when you disturb your circadian rhythm, you also disrupt autophagy. When you get too much exposure to blue light from screens, you disturb your circadian rhythm. When you don't keep a regular and consistent schedule of sleeping and waking times, you disrupt your circadian rhythm.

Sleep affects your physical and emotional well-being. It affects your waking life and can greatly diminish or enhance its quality.

If you don't get the right amount of high-quality sleep, you feel its toll on your emotional balance, productivity, energy, and even your weight.

You don't have to struggle or toss and turn for countless hours before you are able to fall asleep.

You simply have to develop the right habits (affecting both your daytime and bedtime routine) so you are able to sleep better.

Getting the right amount of sleep gives you a lot of health benefits. You become sharp and alert. You are more focused. You have more energy. You are able to keep your emotions on an even keel.

Some simple tips for better sleep include the following:

- Maintain a regular sleeping and waking schedule.

- Get enough sunlight.

- Get enough exercise during the day.

- Limit nicotine and caffeine.

- Avoid sugary snacks, especially at night.

- Don't eat too much at dinner.

- Indulge in a warm bath.

- Turn off all technological gadgets 1 or 2 hours before sleep.

- Avoid blue screens an hour or 2 before your bedtime.

- Dim the lights in your bedroom just before turning in.

- Bring your bedroom's temperature down to 65 degrees.

- Use a sleep app or a sound machine to help you sleep better.

- Wind down through mediation or deep-breathing exercises before sleep.

Fasting

People argue a lot about what food to eat and what food to avoid. Everybody wants to find out what foods promote health and well-being, and which ones increase your risk for heart disease, hypertension, low immunity, and other adverse health conditions.

Unfortunately, people tend to overlook the fact that aside from determining WHAT food to eat, you should also pay serious attention to WHEN you eat. There are convincing indications that when you time your meals intelligently, you are likely to experience significant health benefits.

Fasting is one of the earliest healing strategies used and recommended by philosophers and healers from centuries back.

There are many narrations of fasting in history. Jesus fasted. People still go on fasts today for various reasons. The Christians go on fasts during the Lenten season. The Muslims do it for Ramadan. The Buddhist monks are known to go on fasts on a regular basis.

Fasting seemed to have lost its foothold as a curative and therapeutic strategy when people started using other modern strategies better identified with mainstream medicine.

Fortunately, fasting appears to have made a strong comeback in recent years. It is now widely practiced in the United Kingdom and the United States. People are embracing time-restricted feeding (which has a number of modified forms) and whole day fasting as strategies for improving health.

People are once again taking to fasting as an effective and inexpensive nutritional strategy to reduce inflammation and prevent chronic disease.

Myths about Fasting

Fasting is a powerful tool to improve health. It resets metabolism. It protects your brain. It helps you lose weight.

Fasting reduces bloating, gassiness, and leaky gut. It lowers cholesterol levels and hypertension. It is good for the heart and the liver. It helps reduce insomnia and depression.

You can't ignore the health benefits of fasting.

However, you can't disregard the fact that there are many myths and doubts that surround the concept of fasting. Some individuals hesitate to make fasting part of their lifestyle habits. They seem uncertain whether or not they can safely and effectively integrate fasting into their lives.

These are some of the more common objections to fasting:

- Fasting gets your body into starvation mode.

Fasting is NOT synonymous with starving.

When you fast, you do so deliberately. You do it by choice. You determine when to start and end fasting; you are in control.

A person who starves is not fasting. He simply does not have food. He is not in control as to when his starvation ends.

When your body thinks that it is starving, it goes on survival mode by slowing down metabolism. It holds on to its stored energy by burning fewer calories.

There is actually such a thing as adaptive thermogenesis. When you lose a lot of weight over the long term, your body adapts by reducing the amount of energy it uses. It saves energy by burning fewer calories.

The body uses this adaptive strategy to deal with long-term weight loss – regardless of what method was used to bring about the loss of weight.

There is very little proof to show that the body goes on starvation mode only with intermittent fasting.

In fact, there are studies which indicate that short-term fasts, contrary to what most people believe, can cause the body to increase its metabolic rate.

When you go on short-term fasts, your body releases more norepinephrine, a hormone that stimulates metabolism by telling fat cells to break down fat mass.

When the body is in a fasting state, your metabolism gets a boost. You burn -- not fewer, but more calories.

- Fasting causes muscles to waste.

The body stores and uses sugar as its primary source of energy. During the 24 to 48 hours of fasting, you use sugar (stored as glycogen) for fuel.

When you continue to fast after 48 hours, your body's store of sugar becomes depleted. Your body shifts to using fat as its source of energy. It breaks down the fatty deposits stored in your body and uses it as fuel.

The body does not use protein for fuel. It is wrong to say then that muscles break down when you fast.

- Fasting leads to malnourishment.

When you fast, you refrain from eating to create a calorie deficit.

When you do intermittent fasting, you stop eating (or severely restrict your calorie intake) for between 12 to 24 hours. You will not lose essential vitamins, minerals, and other nutrients or become worn-out, weak, and malnourished.

When you break your fast and eat, you get the nutrients that the body needs.

Intermittent Fasting Strategies

There are many variations of intermittent fasting. If you want to incorporate fasting into your daily lifestyle, you may find it helpful to begin with a short fast. Once you get used to fasting for a few hours, you can then move on to a more challenging fasting schedule.

It is important to start simple and build your way up. This gives your body the time it needs to acclimatize to staying off food at certain times during the day.

You can start with a simple fast. Keep at it for a week or two and observe how your body feels. Using your body's response as basis, you can scale up or down on the number of fasting hours.

1.   Simple Fast

This is the basic fast; it has the shortest duration. Being the easiest to do, it is the strategy recommended for beginners.

The simple fast requires you to go without food for 12 hours. This timeframe includes your sleeping hours.

This strategy allows the liver to purify the bloodstream. It allows the gut to slow down. It triggers the body to burn fat. All these help to activate the drainage pathways and cleanse the system.

How to do it:

Schedule to have dinner early. If you finish eating by 7 pm, refrain from eating again until 7 the next morning.

Continue this schedule for a couple of weeks. After this, extend your fasting hours to 14 hours. If you finish your dinner by 7 pm, don't eat again until 9 the next morning. Maintain the 14-hour fast for 1 to 2 weeks.

2.   Cycle Fast

This is similar to the simple fast with a few challenging modifications. Instead of fasting for 12 to 14 hours, you fast for 16 hours. You don't fast every day. You do it only three times a week.

How to do it:

If you end dinner at 7 pm on Monday, you only get to eat again at 11 am on Tuesday. You don't fast the rest of the time. After your dinner at 7 on Wednesday evening, you go on a 16-hour fast again and have your next meal at 11 am on Thursday. You follow the same cycle during the remaining days of the week. Following this schedule, your fasting days would be Tuesday, Thursday, and Saturday.

You need to do some planning when you go on the cycle fast. This strategy, however, is a good way to prepare you for more advanced and challenging intermittent fasting.

An alternative method would be to continue with the simple fast and just add an hour more of fasting every one or two weeks. This is also a good way to prepare you for the strong fast.

3.   The Strong Fast

This is a more difficult extended form of the simple fast. You fast for between 16 to 18 hours every day.

How to do it:

If you are done with dinner at 7 on Monday evening, you get to eat only at 10 am or 12 noon the next day.

The strong fast is not recommended for beginners. However, an individual who has already gone through intermittent fasting or a keto diet for quite some time is likely to have the metabolic flexibility to successfully go on a strong fast.

Most people who have gone through intermittent fasting for some time say that the strong fast is the sweet spot to aspire for. It gives the most benefits in terms of performance and health.

If you want to achieve optimum energy, try to work towards the strong fast. If you have some health issues you want to address, you may also find it beneficial to work your way up to a strong fast.

4.   Warrior Fast

The warrior fast is considered an extremely demanding and challenging intermittent fasting strategy. Your eating window is limited to 3 to 5 hours only. You fast for 19 to 21 hours.

Few people can handle this strategy. However, those who manage to stick to it say that the strategy comes with extensive benefits.

How to do it:

You finish dinner by 7 on Monday night. Your next meal will be at 1 or 3 pm on Tuesday. You have between 3 to 5 hours to eat and replenish you calorie requirements before you go on a fast again from 7 pm Tuesday until 1 or 3 pm Wednesday.

A modified form of the Warrior Fast is known as Fat Fasting. Technically speaking, the Fat Fast is not really a fast. You get to eat fatty food at any point during your fasting window.

5.   Fat Fasting

This modified strategy supports fat burning and ketosis. It is not fasting in the traditional sense. However, it gives you the same benefits.

How to do it:

Instead of having a meal that contains carbs, fats, and protein to break your fast between 1 and 3 pm, you eat a meal that only has pure fats. For example, you can choose from the following options:

- an ounce of chicken mixed with 2 tablespoons of cream cheese

- 2 egg yolks with a tablespoon of mayonnaise

- ½ small avocado mixed with a tablespoon of mayonnaise

- a cup of Fat-Burning Coffee with ¼ cup of heavy cream blended in

The meal should be low in calories and very high in fat content.

The Fat Fasting strategy helps you reach the condition of ketosis. It also helps prevent hunger pangs which you are likely to experience during the long fasting window.

How Do You Apply these Strategies in Your Daily Life?

Going on long fasts can give you the benefits associated with autophagy. However, you get to enjoy these benefits even if you don't go on a 16-hour fast every day.

You can simply combine intermittent fasting strategies.

- Go on a 24-hour fast once a week.

This method allows you to enjoy the benefits of intermittent fasting without changing your entire weekly eating schedule.

Simply choose a day that is most convenient for you and fast for 24 hours. You can maintain a short fasting window the rest of the week.

Few people can put up with a 16-hour fast every day. However, more people can tolerate going on the longer 24-hour fast once a week.

It is best to do the 24-hour fast on a day that doesn't have a taxing or demanding schedule. For example, many individuals do very well when they fast from Saturday evening to Sunday evening.

- Combine cyclic ketogenic diet with one day of 24-hour fasting and daily short-duration intermittent fasting

Spend Monday through Friday on intermittent fasting and ketogenic meals. On Saturday, you can have higher-carb meal plans. Fast for 24 hours from Saturday night to Sunday night.

- 5:2 Modified Fast

This is a popular strategy. You select 2 days a week where you take in only 500 calories. You can eat normally during the other 5 days.

Nutritionists suggest that you don't do your fasting during two consecutive days. Separate the fasting days with one or more normal-eating days.

The 5:2 Modified Fast has been found to be helpful in reducing fat and improving insulin sensitivity.

- Alternate Day Fasting

You eat on alternate days. On the days when you fast, you are allowed to eat only one meal with a total calorie count of only 500 calories.

If you want to enjoy sustainable weight-loss benefits, you shouldn't go overboard and go on food binges on your eating days. You can eat but within reason.

Fasting on alternate days helps to boost performance in endurance training. It doesn't cause feelings of deprivation; you don't have any unusual food cravings. It helps you lose weight.

- Extended Fasting

Fasting 5 days a month for 3 consecutive months can result in health benefits. It drives cells to regenerate more quickly. It decreases the risk for heart disease, diabetes, gastrointestinal problems, metabolic disorders, and cancer. It improves the immune system. It also delays the signs associated with early aging.

Fasting for more than 48 straight hours is considered extended fasting. People are usually successful with a fasting period of within 3 to 5 days.

During this time, it is prudent to see to it that your stress levels stay low. You should replenish essential minerals by taking trace mineral and salt supplements. You should watch carefully so you immediately notice if your body shows any adverse responses.

If you decide to go on a water fast that lasts for more than 5 days, you should consult your doctor before doing so. Few people are able to hold out without food for this period of time. If you do the fast properly, however, you will enjoy the many health benefits it offers.

Prolonged fasting of this kind should be limited to once or thrice a year.

How to break an Extended Fast

When you go on an extended fast, you have to keep in mind that your digestive system shuts off during this time. You have to break the fast in a gradual and gentle way. If you break your fast by having a large meal, you make your body go through great stress.

If you go on a 3 to 5 day fast, it is best to break your fast in the following manner:

Take only fermented drinks, soups, and broths during the first 1-to-3 days after you break your fast. Bone broth is particularly good because it provides a great deal of nutrients necessary to heal the gut by supporting its mucosal barrier.

Follow the initial 1-to-3 days with light meals and low-carb easy-to-digest smoothies for another 1-3 days.

After this, gradually incorporate small amounts of protein, lightly cooked vegetables, healthy fats, and other easily digestible solid food into your diet.

Challenges Common to Fasting and How to Deal with Them

If you successfully reduce your carb intake and make the shift to a low-carb, high-fat eating plan, you are likely to experience many health benefits.

However, it can be pretty difficult to make the initial shift. You have to deal with certain challenges.

- Unstable Blood Sugar Levels

Your energy level becomes unstable. You have to deal with strong cravings. These difficulties are usually triggered by the blood sugar imbalance brought on by the new nutritional plan.

You can stabilize your blood sugar and diminish cravings by doing the following:

o   Drink water.

o   Eat a small orange or apple. (Stay away from junk food).

o   Get a hot shower.

o   Take a brisk walk. Exercise releases feel-good chemicals or endorphins which help still your cravings.

o   Avoid stress.

o   Get some rest or sleep.

o   Take a multivitamin.

o   Avoid anything that can trigger your cravings

- Adrenal Fatigue

Fasting can trigger adrenal fatigue. Symptoms include body aches, fatigue, low blood pressure, dizziness, unexplained weight loss, skin discoloration, and hair problem.

You can deal with adrenal fatigue by:

o Drinking enough water and drinks with electrolyte minerals

o Doing deep-breathing exercises

o Getting enough sun

o Avoiding stress

o Taking magnesium supplements

o Starting with a simple fast before moving on to strategies with longer fasting windows.

- Constipation

If you are not able to move your bowels regularly, this can reduce the benefits you gain from intermittent fasting.

Constipation is also harmful. It allows waste to accumulate and decay in the colon. It creates toxins that get into the blood stream and cause inflammation. It slows down brain function.

Prevent constipation by doing the following:

o Take a lot of water. Take liquids with some salt.

o Take magnesium supplements.

o Include fiber-rich food like avocado, onions, garlic, cruciferous vegetables, and leafy veggies in your diet.

o Drink tea.

o Take aloe vera and other herbs recognized for promoting regular bowel movement.

o   Take probiotics for better bowel dynamics.

Conclusion

I'd like to thank you and congratulate you for transiting my lines from start to finish.

I hope this book was able to help you to appreciate autophagy and the many positive things it does to promote health.

Now that you understand how autophagy works, the next step is to apply one or more of the various autophagy strategies discussed.

Start easy. Go on a simple fast. Once you get used to it, you can start working your way up. If you want to enjoy the highest level of autophagy benefits, you can use fasting in combination with a keto lifestyle. You will soon see an amazing improvement in your health, as well as in your sense of well-being. Use the principles of autophagy to bring you closer to achieving all your health and wellness goals.

I wish you the best of luck!

Free Stuff

Do you want to get notified when I have free books? Then sign up for my newsletter. I will never spam you. I will only send you valuable stuff that you can use to help you improve your life.

Sign up here - http://forms.aweber.com/form/26/1968511626.htm

www.ingramcontent.com/pod-product-compliance
Lightning Source LLC
Chambersburg PA
CBHW032104280526
45784CB00013B/3139